Copyright 2023

All right reserved. No part of this book should be resproduce without express permission of the author.

Reproduction of all or any part of this book is punishable under relevant law.

Table of Contents

A blockage of blood flow to the heart muscle.

A heart attack is a medical emergency. A heart attack usually occurs when a blood clot blocks blood flow to the heart. Without blood, tissue loses oxygen and dies.

Symptoms include tightness or pain in the chest, neck, back or arms, as well as fatigue, lightheadedness, abnormal heartbeat and anxiety. Women are more likely to have atypical symptoms than men.

Treatment ranges from lifestyle changes and cardiac rehabilitation to medication, stents and bypass surgery.

BREAKFAST

1. Chocolate Muffins

Prep Time: 15 Minutes

Cook Time: 1hrs 5 Minutes

Servings: 12

Ingredients

- ¾ cup all-purpose flour
- ¾ cup whole-wheat flour
- ¾ cup granulated sugar
- ¾ cup cocoa powder
- 1 teaspoon instant espresso powder
- 1 teaspoon baking soda
- ¼ teaspoon salt
- 2 large eggs, at room temperature
- ¾ cup whole-milk plain yogurt
- ½ cup canola oil or other neutral oil
- ½ cup low-fat buttermilk
- 2 teaspoons vanilla extract

- ¼ cup dark chocolate chips (60-70% cacao)

Instructions

1. Preheat oven to 425°F. Coat a 12-cup muffin tin with cooking spray and line with paper liners.
2. Whisk all-purpose flour, whole-wheat flour, sugar, cocoa, espresso powder, baking soda and salt together in a large bowl until combined and free of lumps.
3. Whisk eggs, yogurt, oil, buttermilk and vanilla together in a medium bowl until combined. Gently stir the egg mixture into the flour mixture until just combined. Pour the batter evenly into the prepared muffin cups (heaping 1/4 cup each). Sprinkle the tops evenly with chocolate chips.
4. Bake for 5 minutes. Reduce oven temperature to 350°F (do not remove muffins from oven). Bake until a wooden pick inserted in the center of the muffins comes out clean, 15 to 20 minutes. Let the muffins cool in the pan for 10 minutes. Turn out onto a wire rack and cool for about 15 more minutes. Serve warm or at room temperature.

Prep Time: 10 Minutes

Cook Time: 40 Minutes

Servings: 2

Ingredients

- 1 medium sweet potato, scrubbed and sliced into 1/2-inch rounds
- 2 teaspoons extra-virgin olive oil
- ½ teaspoon ground cumin
- ¼ teaspoon salt, divided
- ½ avocado
- 1 tablespoon salsa
- 1 tablespoon finely chopped red onion
- 2 whole-grain English muffins, toasted
- 2 large eggs, fried
- ½ cup baby spinach leaves

Instructions

1. Preheat oven to 400°F.

2. Toss sweet potato slices with oil, cumin and 1/8 teaspoon salt. Arrange in a single layer on a large rimmed baking sheet. Roast, turning once, until tender, 25 to 30 minutes. Reserve 2 slices about the size of the English muffins. Save the other slices for another use.

3. Meanwhile, mash avocado, salsa, red onion and remaining 1/8 teaspoon salt together on a small plate.

4. Spread half of the avocado mixture on 1 English muffin half. Top with a sweet potato round, an egg and 1/4 cup spinach. Place the remaining muffin half on top. Repeat with the remaining ingredients.

Prep Time: 30Minutes

Cook Time: 30Minutes

Servings: 4

Ingredients

- 1 tablespoon extra-virgin olive oil
- ½ cup chopped onion
- 3 cups chopped cauliflower
- ½ cup chopped red bell pepper
- ½ teaspoon dried marjoram
- ¼ teaspoon salt
- ¼ teaspoon ground pepper
- 2 tablespoons pesto
- 4 slices whole-grain country bread, toasted
- 1 ¼ cups shredded extra-sharp Cheddar cheese

Instruction

1. Heat oil in a large skillet over medium heat. Add onion; cook, stirring, until starting to soften, about 3 minutes. Add cauliflower, bell pepper, marjoram, salt and

pepper; cook, stirring, until the vegetables are tender, 6 to 8 minutes more. Add pesto and stir to coat. Remove from heat.

2. Position rack in upper third of oven; preheat broiler to high.

3. Place toasted bread on a baking sheet and divide the vegetable mixture among the toasts. Top each with about 1/4 cup cheese. Broil until the cheese is melted and browned in spots, about 3 minutes.

Prep Time: 10 Minutes

Cook Time: 10 Mnutes

Servings: 1

Ingredients

- 2 tablespoons whole-wheat pastry flour
- 1 tablespoon cocoa powder
- 1 tablespoon light brown sugar
- ⅛ Teaspoon baking soda
- Pinch of salt
- 1 tablespoon low-fat milk
- 1 tablespoon water
- 2 teaspoons canola oil
- 2 teaspoons crunchy natural peanut butter
- ⅛ Teaspoon vanilla extract
- Unsalted roasted peanuts, bittersweet chocolate chips and/or coarse sea salt (optional)

Instructions

1. Coat a 12- to 16-ounce microwaveable mug with cooking spray.
2. Whisk flour, cocoa, brown sugar, baking soda and salt together in a small bowl. Add milk, water, oil, peanut butter and vanilla; stir until smooth.
3. Pour the mixture into the prepared mug. Sprinkle the top with peanuts, chocolate chips and/or sea salt, if desired. Microwave on High until the cake doubles in size, 30 to 45 seconds. Serve immediately.

Prep Time: 20 Minutes

Cook Time: 4hrs 20 Minutes

Servings: 6

Ingredients

- 1 ½ cups dried chickpeas, soaked overnight
- 4 cups water
- 1 large yellow onion, finely chopped
- 1 (15 ounce) can no-salt-added diced tomatoes, preferably fire-roasted
- 2 tablespoons tomato paste
- 4 cloves garlic, finely chopped
- 1 bay leaf
- 4 teaspoons ground cumin
- 4 teaspoons paprika
- ¼ teaspoon cayenne pepper
- ¼ teaspoon ground pepper
- 2 pounds bone-in chicken thighs, skin removed, trimmed
- 1 (14 ounce) can artichoke hearts, drained and quartered

- ¼ cup halved pitted oil-cured olives
- ½ teaspoon salt
- ¼ cup chopped fresh parsley or cilantro

Instructions

1. Gather all the ingredients.
2. Drain 1 1/2 cups chickpeas and place in a 6-quart or larger slow cooker. Add 4 cups water, onion, tomatoes and their juice, 2 tablespoons tomato paste, garlic, bay leaf, 4 teaspoons cumin, 4 teaspoon paprika, 1/4 teaspoon cayenne and 1/4 teaspoon ground pepper; stir to combine. Add 2 pounds chicken. Cover and cook on Low for 8 hours or High for 4 hours.
3. Transfer the chicken to a clean cutting board and let cool slightly. Discard bay leaf. Add artichokes, 1/4 cup olives and 1/2 teaspoon salt to the slow cooker and stir to combine.
4. Shred the chicken, discarding bones. Stir the chicken into the soup.
5. Serve topped with 1/4 cup parsley (or cilantro).

Prep Time: 15 Minutes

Cook Time: 30 Mnutes

Servings: 4

Ingredients

- 1/2 cup coarse dry breadcrumbs, preferably whole-wheat
- 1 tablespoon extra-virgin olive oil
- 1 tablespoon whole-grain mustard
- 1 tablespoon chopped shallot
- 1 tablespoon lemon juice
- 1 teaspoon chopped rinsed capers
- 1 teaspoon chopped fresh thyme, or 1/2 teaspoon dried
- 1 ¼ pounds center-cut salmon fillet, skinned and cut lengthwise into 4 strips
- 4 teaspoons low-fat mayonnaise

Instructions

1. Preheat oven to 400 degrees F. Coat a 9-by-13-inch baking dish with cooking spray.

2. Mix breadcrumbs, oil, mustard, shallot, lemon juice, capers and thyme in a small bowl until combined.

3. Working with one at a time, spread each salmon strip with 1 teaspoon mayonnaise. Spread about 3 tablespoons of the breadcrumb mixture over the mayonnaise. Starting at one end, roll the salmon up tightly, tucking in any loose filling as you go. Insert a toothpick though the end to keep the pinwheel from unrolling. Place in the prepared dish. Repeat with the remaining salmon strips.

4. Bake the pinwheels until just cooked through, 15 to 20 minutes. Remove the toothpicks before serving.

Prep Time: 40 Minutes

Cook Time: 1hrs 15 Minutes

Servings: 8

Ingredients

- 1 medium head cauliflower, cut into small florets
- 1 medium zucchini, cut into small cubes
- 1 medium red bell pepper, cut into small cubes
- 2 tablespoons extra-virgin olive oil
- 1 teaspoon dried oregano
- ¾ teaspoon salt, divided
- ½ teaspoon ground pepper, divided
- 1 pound ziti
- 1 (24 ounce) jar lower-sodium marinara sauce
- 1 cup part-skim ricotta cheese
- ½ cup grated Parmesan cheese
- ¼ cup chopped fresh flat-leaf parsley
- 2 cups shredded low-moisture part-skim mozzarella cheese

Instructions

1. Position rack in lower third of oven; preheat to 450°F. Coat a 9-by-13-inch baking dish with cooking spray.

2. Toss cauliflower, zucchini, bell pepper, oil and oregano together in a large bowl. Sprinkle with 1/4 teaspoon each salt and pepper; toss again to mix. Spread the mixture in an even layer on a large rimmed baking sheet. Roast the vegetables until slightly charred and tender, about 20 minutes. Remove from the oven and set aside. Do not turn the oven off.

3. Meanwhile, bring a large pot of water to a boil over medium-high heat. Add ziti and cook according to package directions. Drain the ziti and transfer to a large heatproof bowl.

4. Add the roasted vegetables, marinara and the remaining 1/2 teaspoon salt and 1/4 teaspoon pepper to the ziti in the bowl. Toss well to coat. Spread the mixture evenly in the prepared baking dish.

5. Stir ricotta, Parmesan and parsley together in a small bowl. Add spoonfuls of the ricotta mixture to the pasta mixture in the baking dish and gently stir to loosely combine. Sprinkle the mixture evenly with mozzarella. Bake at 450°F until the casserole is bubbly and the

cheese is melted and slightly browned, about 25 minutes. Let stand for 5 minutes before serving.

Prep Time: 15 Minutes

Cook Time: 2hrs 20 Minutes

Servings: 8

Ingredients

- 1 (15 ounce) can tomato puree
- 1 (4 ounce) can chopped green chiles, undrained
- 1 small sweet onion, finely chopped (about 1/2 cup)
- 1 cup water
- ⅓ Cup packed light brown sugar
- ⅓ Cup cider vinegar
- 2 tablespoons tomato paste
- 1 tablespoon dry mustard
- 1 teaspoon Worcestershire sauce
- 1 teaspoon smoked paprika
- ½ teaspoon garlic powder
- ½ teaspoon onion powder
- ½ teaspoon ground pepper
- ¼ teaspoon salt
- 1 (2 pound) pork tenderloin, trimmed

Instructions

1. Combine tomato puree, green chiles, onion, water, brown sugar, vinegar, tomato paste, mustard, Worcestershire, paprika, garlic powder, onion powder, pepper and salt in a 6-quart slow cooker; stir until combined.

2. If needed, cut pork in half crosswise to fit inside the cooker. Add the pork to the sauce in the cooker; stir to coat. Cover and cook, flipping once, until a thermometer inserted into the thickest portion registers 145°F, 2 hours to 2 hours, 30 minutes on High or 3 to 4 hours on Low. Transfer the pork to a plate; cover with foil and let rest for 10 minutes.

3. Meanwhile, use an immersion blender to puree the sauce in the slow cooker until smooth, about 1 minute. (Use caution when blending hot liquids.)

4. Slice the pork into 1/2-inch-thick slices. Pour half of the sauce (about 2 cups) over the pork before serving. (Save any remaining sauce for another use.)

Prep Time: 1hrs 5 Minutes

Cook Time: 2hrs 2 Minutes

Servings: 6

Ingredients

- 8 ounces whole-wheat egg noodles
- 1 cup sliced fresh asparagus
- 2 tablespoons extra-virgin olive oil plus 1 teaspoon, divided
- 1 medium leek, halved lengthwise and thinly sliced crosswise
- 2 teaspoons minced garlic
- ¼ cup all-purpose flour
- 3 ½ cups whole milk
- 1 tablespoon Dijon mustard
- ½ teaspoon salt
- ½ teaspoon ground pepper
- ¼ teaspoon cayenne pepper
- 2 (6 ounce) cans no-salt-added boneless, skinless pink salmon, drained and flaked
- 1 cup frozen peas, thawed

- ½ cup whole-wheat panko breadcrumbs
- ½ cup shredded white Cheddar cheese
- 1 tablespoon finely chopped fresh flat-leaf parsley

Instructions

1. Preheat oven to 375°F. Bring a large pot of water to a boil over high heat. Add noodles; cook, stirring occasionally, until slightly softened but still somewhat firm, about 5 minutes (the noodles will be undercooked). Add asparagus; cook, stirring often, until the asparagus is bright green and tender-crisp and the noodles are fully cooked, about 2 minutes. Drain and set aside.

2. Wipe the pot clean. Add 2 tablespoons oil and heat over medium-high heat. Add leek; cook, stirring occasionally, until softened and translucent, about 5 minutes. Add garlic; cook, stirring often, until fragrant, about 1 minute. Sprinkle with flour. Reduce heat to medium and cook, stirring constantly, for 2 minutes. Gradually add milk, whisking until smooth. Bring to a gentle boil over medium-high heat, whisking often. Reduce heat to medium-low; gently simmer, whisking often, until thickened, about 5 minutes. Remove from

heat. Add mustard, salt, pepper and cayenne; stir until well combined. Add the noodle-asparagus mixture, salmon and peas; fold until the noodles are fully coated. Spread the mixture evenly in a 2-quart baking dish.

3. Combine panko, cheese, parsley and the remaining 1 teaspoon oil in a medium bowl; stir until well mixed. Sprinkle evenly over the casserole. Bake until the cheese is melted and the topping is golden brown, about 15 minutes. Let stand for 5 minutes before serving.

Prep Time: 30 Minutes

Cook Time: 30 Mnutes

Servings: 12

Ingredients

- 2 tablespoons extra-virgin olive oil
- 4 bell peppers, sliced
- 3 cups sliced sweet onions
- 1 teaspoon salt

Instructions

1. Heat oil in a large straight-sided sauté pan or Dutch oven over medium heat. Add peppers, onions and salt; cook, stirring occasionally, until the vegetables are tender and starting to brown, 18 to 21 minutes.

11. Butternut Squash Casserole

Prep Time: 1hrs 5 Minutes

Cook Time: 2hrs 10 Minutes

Servings: 10

Ingredients

- 2 (2 pound) butternut squash, halved lengthwise and seeded
- 1 tablespoon extra-virgin olive oil
- ½ cup old-fashioned rolled oats
- ½ cup chopped pecans
- ¾ cup light brown sugar, divided
- ¼ cup unsalted butter, melted, divided
- ½ cup whole milk
- 2 large eggs, lightly beaten
- 1 teaspoon cornstarch
- 1 teaspoon salt
- ½ teaspoon ground cinnamon

Instructions

1. Preheat oven to 400°F. Line a rimmed baking sheet with foil or parchment paper. Rub squash halves evenly with oil; arrange, cut-side down, on the prepared baking sheet. Bake until very tender, about 45 minutes. Let cool for about 20 minutes. Reduce oven temperature to 350°F.

2. While the squash cools, lightly coat a 9-inch-square baking dish with cooking spray; set aside. Combine oats, pecans, 1/4 cup brown sugar and 2 tablespoons melted butter in a medium bowl; set aside.

3. Scoop the squash flesh into a large bowl; discard shells. Mash the squash with a fork until smooth. Stir in milk, eggs, cornstarch, salt, cinnamon and the remaining 1/2 cup brown sugar and 2 tablespoons melted butter. Spoon the mixture into the prepared baking dish; sprinkle evenly with the oat mixture. Bake until golden and set, about 35 minutes. Let stand for 15 minutes before serving.

Prep Time: 50 Minutes

Cook Time: 50 Minutes

Servings: 4

Ingredients

- 4 tablespoons extra-virgin olive oil, divided
- 1 cup diced shallots
- ½ cup diced celery
- 5 cups sliced shiitake mushroom caps (about 10 ounces), divided
- 5 cups sliced baby bella mushrooms (about 10 ounces), divided
- ½ cup dry sherry
- 3 cloves garlic, minced
- 4 cups diced peeled Yukon Gold potatoes (about 1 pound)
- ½ teaspoon dried thyme
- 3 cups "no-chicken broth" or mushroom broth
- 1 cup water
- ½ cup walnuts, finely chopped
- Pinch of salt

- 2 teaspoons sherry vinegar
- ½ teaspoon ground pepper
- 2 tablespoons sliced fresh chives

Instructions

1. Heat 3 tablespoons oil in a large pot over medium heat. Add shallots and celery; cook, stirring occasionally, until tender, about 3 minutes. Add 4 cups each shiitakes and baby bellas, sherry and garlic; cook, stirring occasionally, until the mushrooms are soft and the liquid has evaporated, about 5 minutes. Stir in potatoes and thyme; cook for 1 minute. Add broth and water. Bring to a boil. Reduce heat to maintain a simmer and cook, stirring occasionally, until the vegetables are very soft, about 20 minutes.

2. Meanwhile, coarsely chop the remaining 2 cups mushrooms. Heat the remaining 1 tablespoon oil in a medium skillet over medium heat. Add the mushrooms and cook, stirring often, until soft, about 2 minutes. Add walnuts and salt. Cook, stirring occasionally, until hot, about 1 minute more.

3. Puree the soup with an immersion blender or in a regular blender (in batches, if necessary) until very

smooth. (Use caution when blending hot liquids.) Stir in vinegar and pepper.

4. Serve the soup topped with the mushroom-walnut mixture and chives.

Prep Time: 15 Minutes

Cook Time: 35 Minutes

Servings: 4

Ingredients

- 2 tablespoons extra-virgin olive oil, divided
- 4 large bone-in chicken thighs, skin removed
- ½ teaspoon garlic powder
- ½ teaspoon salt, divided
- ½ teaspoon ground pepper, divided
- 1 medium onion, halved and thinly sliced
- ½ cup low-sodium chicken broth
- ⅓ cup balsamic vinegar
- 1 tablespoon honey

Instructions

1. Heat 1 tablespoon oil in a large skillet over medium-high heat. Season chicken all over with garlic powder and 1/4 teaspoon each salt and pepper. Cook the

chicken, turning once, until well browned on both sides, 6 to 8 minutes total. Transfer to a plate.

2. Lower heat to medium and add the remaining 1 tablespoon oil and onions to the pan. Cook, stirring, until mostly softened, about 4 minutes. Add broth, vinegar, honey and the remaining 1/4 teaspoon each salt and pepper; whisk to combine. Return the chicken to the pan, partially cover and cook, turning once, until the liquid has reduced and an instant-read thermometer inserted in the thickest part without touching the bone registers 165°F, 10 to 15 minutes.

Prep Time: 35 Minutes

Cook Time: 35 Minutes

Servings: 8

Ingredients

- 2 tablespoons extra-virgin olive oil
- 1 10-ounce bag frozen seasoning blend thawed
- 3 cloves garlic, thinly sliced
- 1 ½ teaspoons smoked paprika
- 4 cups lower-sodium vegetable broth
- 2 cups water
- 1 (14.5 ounce) can fire-roasted diced tomatoes, undrained
- 1 medium head green cabbage, cored and chopped
- 3 small Yukon Gold potatoes, peeled and chopped
- 2 tablespoons chopped fresh thyme, plus more for garnish
- ¾ teaspoon salt
- 2 tablespoons plus 2 teaspoons lemon juice
- Lemon wedges for serving

Instructions

1. Heat oil in a large Dutch oven or other large heavy pot over medium-high heat. Add seasoning blend; cook, stirring occasionally, until tender, about 5 minutes. Add garlic and paprika; cook, stirring constantly, until fragrant, about 30 seconds. Stir in broth, water, tomatoes, cabbage, potatoes, thyme and salt; bring to a boil over high heat. Reduce heat to medium-low; cover and simmer, stirring occasionally, until the cabbage and potatoes are tender, about 25 minutes. Remove from heat and divide among 8 bowls; stir in 1 teaspoon lemon juice per bowl. Garnish with additional thyme, if desired, and serve with lemon wedges.

Prep Time: 20 Minutes

Cook Time: 40 Minutes

Servings: 10

Ingredients

- 2 tablespoons extra-virgin olive oil
- 8 ounces mushrooms, sliced (2 1/2 cups)
- ½ cup sliced shallots
- 4 cups frozen cut green beans
- 2 cups low-sodium vegetable broth or "no-chicken" broth
- 3/4-1 cup plain unsweetened almond milk
- ¼ cup all-purpose flour
- 1 tablespoon reduced-sodium soy sauce
- 1 teaspoon ground pepper
- ½ teaspoon salt
- 1 cup Vegan French-Fried Onions

Instructions

1. Preheat oven to 375 degrees F. Heat oil in a large pot over medium-high heat. Add mushrooms and shallots. Cook, stirring frequently, until the mushrooms have released their liquid, 4 to 6 minutes.

2. Add green beans and broth and bring to a boil. Whisk 3/4 cup almond milk and flour together in a medium bowl. Add to the green bean mixture and cook, stirring, until bubbling and thickened, 2 to 3 minutes. If the sauce seems too thick, add an additional 1/4 cup almond milk. Stir in soy sauce, pepper and salt. Transfer the mixture to a 9-by-13-inch baking dish.

3. Sprinkle french-fried onions over the top of the casserole. Bake until bubbling and the onions are golden brown, 20 to 25 minutes.

Prep Time: 30 Minutes

Cook Time: 30 Minutes

Servings: 4

Ingredients

- 1 bunch scallions
- ¼ cup lower-sodium soy sauce
- 2 tablespoons mirin
- 2 tablespoons dark brown sugar
- 3 teaspoons cornstarch, divided
- ¾ teaspoon ground pepper, divided
- 4 (4 ounce) boneless, skinless chicken thighs, cut into bite-size pieces
- 2 tablespoons vegetable oil, divided
- 4 cups broccoli florets
- 1 medium red bell pepper, thinly sliced
- 1 tablespoon grated fresh ginger
- 2 cups hot cooked brown rice
- Toasted sesame seeds for garnish

Instructions

1. Cut white and light green parts of scallions into 2-inch pieces and set aside in a small bowl. Thinly slice the remaining dark green parts of the scallions and reserve for topping.

2. Combine soy sauce, mirin, brown sugar, 2 teaspoons cornstarch and 1/2 teaspoon pepper in a small bowl; set aside. Toss chicken with the remaining 1 teaspoon cornstarch and 1/4 teaspoon pepper in a large bowl.

3. Heat 1 tablespoon oil in a large nonstick skillet over medium-high heat. Add the chicken; cook, stirring occasionally, until golden brown and cooked through, about 5 minutes. Transfer to a plate.

4. Heat the remaining 1 tablespoon oil in the skillet over medium-high heat. Add broccoli, bell pepper and 2-inch scallion pieces; cook, stirring often, until the vegetables are tender-crisp, about 2 minutes. Return the chicken to the pan and stir in ginger and the reserved soy sauce mixture. Cook, stirring often, until the sauce thickens and coats the chicken, 4 to 5 minutes.

5. Divide rice evenly among 4 bowls. Top with the chicken and vegetable mixture and the reserved sliced scallions; garnish with sesame seeds, if desired.

Prep Time: 10 Minutes

Cook Time: 25 Minutes

Servings: 6

Ingredients

- 2 (15 ounce) cans no-salt-added great northern beans, rinsed, divided
- 1 tablespoon canola oil
- 1 pound boneless, skinless chicken thighs, trimmed and cut into bite-size pieces
- 1 ½ cups chopped yellow onion (1 medium)
- ¾ cup chopped celery (2 medium stalks)
- 5 cloves garlic, chopped (2 tablespoons)
- 1 teaspoon ground cumin
- ¼ teaspoon salt
- 3 cups unsalted chicken stock
- 1 (4 ounce) can chopped green chiles
- 4 ounces reduced-fat cream cheese
- ½ cup loosely packed fresh cilantro leaves

Instructions

1. Mash 1 cup beans in a small bowl with a whisk or potato masher.

2. Heat oil in a large heavy pot over high heat. Add chicken; cook, turning occasionally, until browned, 4 to 5 minutes. Add onion, celery, garlic, cumin and salt. Cook until the onion is translucent and tender, 4 to 5 minutes.

3. Add the remaining whole beans, the mashed beans, stock and chiles. Bring to a boil. Reduce heat to medium and simmer until the chicken is cooked through, about 3 minutes. Remove from heat; stir in cream cheese until melted. Serve topped with cilantro.

Prep Time: 20 Minutes

Cook Time: 40 Minutes

Servings: 4

Ingredients

- 2 teaspoons chili powder
- 2 teaspoons ground cumin
- ¾ teaspoon salt, divided
- ½ teaspoon garlic powder
- ½ teaspoon smoked paprika
- ¼ teaspoon ground pepper
- 2 tablespoons olive oil, divided
- 1 ¼ pounds chicken tenders
- 1 medium yellow onion, sliced
- 1 medium red bell pepper, sliced
- 1 medium green bell pepper, sliced
- 4 cups chopped stemmed kale
- 1 (15 ounce) can no-salt-added black beans, rinsed
- ¼ cup low-fat plain Greek yogurt
- 1 tablespoon lime juice
- 2 teaspoons water

Instructions

1. Place a large rimmed baking sheet in the oven; preheat to 425 degrees F.

2. Combine chili powder, cumin, 1/2 tsp. salt, garlic powder, paprika, and ground pepper in a large bowl. Transfer 1 tsp. of the spice mixture to a medium bowl and set aside. Whisk 1 Tbsp. oil into the remaining spice mixture in the large bowl. Add chicken, onion, and red and green bell peppers; toss to coat.

3. Remove the pan from the oven; coat with cooking spray. Spread the chicken mixture in an even layer on the pan. Roast for 15 minutes.

4. Meanwhile, combine kale and black beans with the remaining 1/4 tsp. salt and 1 Tbsp. olive oil in a large bowl; toss to coat.

5. Remove the pan from the oven. Stir the chicken and vegetables. Spread kale and beans evenly over the top. Roast until the chicken is cooked through and the vegetables are tender, 5 to 7 minutes more.

6. Meanwhile, add yogurt, lime juice, and water to the reserved spice mixture; stir to combine.

7. Divide the chicken and vegetable mixture among 4 bowls. Drizzle with the yogurt dressing and serve.

Prep Time: 16 Minutes

Cook Time: 25 Minutes

Servings: 2

Ingredients

- 4 ounces salmon, preferably wild
- 1 teaspoon avocado oil
- ⅛ teaspoon kosher salt
- 1 cup instant brown rice
- 1 cup water
- 2 tablespoons mayonnaise
- 1 ½ teaspoons Sriracha
- 1 ½ teaspoons 50%-less-sodium tamari
- 1 teaspoon mirin
- ½ teaspoon freshly grated ginger
- ¼ teaspoon crushed red pepper
- ⅛ teaspoon kosher salt
- ½ ripe avocado, chopped
- ½ cup chopped cucumber
- ¼ cup spicy kimchi
- 12 (4-inch) sheets nori (roasted seaweed)

Instructions

1. Preheat oven to 400°F. Line a small rimmed baking sheet with foil. Place salmon on the prepared pan. Drizzle with oil; season with salt. Bake until an instant-read thermometer inserted in the thickest part registers 125°F, 8 to 10 minutes.

2. Meanwhile, combine rice and water in a small saucepan; cook according to package directions. Mix mayonnaise and Sriracha in a small bowl; set aside. Whisk tamari, mirin, ginger, crushed red pepper and salt in another small bowl; set aside.

3. Divide the rice between 2 bowls. Top with salmon, avocado, cucumber and kimchi. Drizzle with the tamari mixture and the mayonnaise mixture. Mix the bowls, if desired, and serve with nori.

Prep Time: 40 Minutes

Cook Time: 4hrs 5 Minutes

Servings: 8

Ingredients

- 1 tablespoon kosher salt
- 2 teaspoons ground cinnamon
- ½ teaspoon ground allspice
- ½ teaspoon ground pepper
- ¼ teaspoon ground cloves
- 3-3 1/2 pounds beef chuck roast, trimmed
- 2 tablespoons extra-virgin olive oil
- 1 medium onion, chopped
- 3 cloves garlic, sliced
- 1 cup red wine
- 1 (28 ounce) can whole tomatoes, preferably San Marzano
- 5 medium carrots, cut into 1-inch pieces
- 2 medium turnips, peeled and cut into 1/2-inch pieces
- Chopped fresh basil for garnish

Instructions

1. Combine salt, cinnamon, allspice, pepper and cloves in a small bowl. Rub the mixture all over beef.

2. Heat oil in a large skillet over medium heat. Add the beef and cook until browned, 4 to 5 minutes per side. Transfer to a 5- to 6-quart slow cooker.

3. Add onion and garlic to the pan. Cook, stirring, for 2 minutes. Add wine and tomatoes (with their juice); bring to a boil, scraping up any browned bits and breaking up the tomatoes. Add the mixture to the slow cooker along with carrots and turnips.

4. Cover and cook on High for 4 hours or Low for 8 hours.

5. Remove the beef from the slow cooker and slice. Serve the beef with the sauce and vegetables, garnished with basil, if desired.

21. Lemon-Garlic Pasta with Salmon

Prep Time: 15 Minutes

Cook Time: 15 Minutes

Servings: 4

Ingredients

- 8 ounces whole-wheat pasta
- 5 tablespoons extra-virgin olive oil
- 5 cloves garlic, chopped
- 1 teaspoon anchovy paste
- ¼ teaspoon crushed red pepper
- Zest and juice of 1 lemon
- 1 1/2 cups flaked cooked salmon
- 3 tablespoons chopped fresh parsley
- ¼ teaspoon salt
- 2 tablespoons whole-wheat breadcrumbs, toasted

Instructions

1. Cook pasta according to package directions. Drain, reserving 1/2 cup cooking water.

2. Combine oil, garlic, anchovy paste, crushed red pepper, lemon zest and lemon juice in a large skillet. Heat over medium-high heat until sizzling, about 3 minutes. Add the reserved water, the pasta, salmon, parsley and salt. Cook, stirring, until the sauce coats the pasta, about 2 minutes. Serve topped with breadcrumbs.

Prep Time: 10 Minutes

Cook Time: 15 Minutes

Servings: 6

Ingredients

- 2 teaspoons extra-virgin olive oil
- 2 leeks, white and light green parts only, cut into 1/4-inch rounds
- 1 tablespoon chopped fresh sage, or 1/4 teaspoon dried
- 2 14-ounce cans reduced-sodium chicken broth
- 2 cups water
- 1 15-ounce can cannellini beans, rinsed
- 1 2-poundi roasted chicken, skin discarded, meat removed from bones and shredded (4 cups)

Instructions

1. Heat oil in a Dutch oven over medium-high heat. Add leeks and cook, stirring often, until soft, about 3 minutes. Stir in sage and continue cooking until aromatic, about 30 seconds. Stir in broth and water,

increase heat to high, cover and bring to a boil. Add beans and chicken and cook, uncovered, stirring occasionally, until heated through, about 3 minutes. Serve hot.

Prep Time: 25 Minutes

Cook Time: 25 Minutes

Servings: 4

Ingredients

- ⅓ cup prepared pesto
- 2 tablespoons balsamic vinegar
- 1 tablespoon extra-virgin olive oil
- ½ teaspoon salt
- ¼ teaspoon ground pepper
- 1 pound peeled and deveined large shrimp (16-20 count), patted dry
- 4 cups arugula
- 2 cups cooked quinoa
- 1 cup halved cherry tomatoes
- 1 avocado, diced

Instructions

1. Whisk pesto, vinegar, oil, salt and pepper in a large
    bowl. Remove 4 tablespoons of the mixture to a small
    bowl; set both bowls aside.
2. Heat a large cast-iron skillet over medium-high heat.
    Add shrimp and cook, stirring, until just cooked
    through with a slight char, 4 to 5 minutes. Remove to a
    plate.
3. Add arugula and quinoa to the large bowl with the
    vinaigrette and toss to coat. Divide the arugula mixture
    between 4 bowls. Top with tomatoes, avocado and
    shrimp. Drizzle each bowl with 1 tablespoon of the
    reserved pesto mixture.

Prep Time: 25 Minutes

Cook Time: 25 Minutes

Servings: 4

Ingredients

- 8 ounces gluten-free penne pasta or whole-wheat penne pasta
- 2 tablespoons extra-virgin olive oil
- 1 pound boneless, skinless chicken breast or thighs, trimmed, if necessary, and cut into bite-size pieces
- ½ teaspoon salt
- ¼ teaspoon ground pepper
- 4 cloves garlic, minced
- ½ cup dry white wine
- Juice and zest of 1 lemon
- 10 cups chopped fresh spinach
- 4 tablespoons grated Parmesan cheese, divided

Instructions

1. Cook pasta according to package directions. Drain and set aside.

2. Meanwhile, heat oil in a large high-sided skillet over medium-high heat. Add chicken, salt and pepper; cook, stirring occasionally, until just cooked through, 5 to 7 minutes. Add garlic and cook, stirring, until fragrant, about 1 minute. Stir in wine, lemon juice and zest; bring to a simmer.

3. Remove from heat. Stir in spinach and the cooked pasta. Cover and let stand until the spinach is just wilted. Divide among 4 plates and top each serving with 1 tablespoon Parmesan.

Prep Time: 10 Minutes

Cook Time: 20 Minutes

Servings: 4

Ingredients

- 2 teaspoons Dijon mustard
- 1 clove garlic, minced
- ¼ teaspoon lemon zest
- 1 teaspoon lemon juice
- 1 teaspoon chopped fresh rosemary
- ½ teaspoon honey
- ½ teaspoon kosher salt
- ¼ teaspoon crushed red pepper
- 3 tablespoons panko breadcrumbs
- 3 tablespoons finely chopped walnuts
- 1 teaspoon extra-virgin olive oil
- 1 (1 pound) skinless salmon fillet, fresh or frozen
- Olive oil cooking spray
- Chopped fresh parsley and lemon wedges for garnish

Instructions

1. Preheat oven to 425 degrees F. Line a large rimmed baking sheet with parchment paper.
2. Combine mustard, garlic, lemon zest, lemon juice, rosemary, honey, salt and crushed red pepper in a small bowl. Combine panko, walnuts and oil in another small bowl.
3. Place salmon on the prepared baking sheet. Spread the mustard mixture over the fish and sprinkle with the panko mixture, pressing to adhere. Lightly coat with cooking spray.
4. Bake until the fish flakes easily with a fork, about 8 to 12 minutes, depending on thickness.
5. Sprinkle with parsley and serve with lemon wedges, if desired.

Prep Time: 35 Minutes

Cook Time: 40 Minutes

Servings: 5

Ingredients

- 8 ounces whole-wheat linguine or spaghetti
- 1 pound boneless, skinless chicken thighs
- 4 cups sliced mushrooms
- 2 cups sliced Brussels sprouts
- 1 medium onion, chopped
- 4 cloves garlic, thinly sliced
- 2 tablespoons Boursin cheese
- 1 ¼ teaspoons dried thyme
- ¾ teaspoon dried rosemary
- ¾ teaspoon salt
- 4 cups water
- 2 tablespoons chopped fresh chives

Instructions

1. Combine pasta, chicken, mushrooms, Brussels sprouts, onion, garlic, Boursin cheese, thyme, rosemary and salt in a large pot. Stir in water. Bring to a boil over high heat. Boil, stirring frequently, until the pasta is cooked and the water has almost evaporated, 10 to 12 minutes. Remove from heat and let stand, stirring occasionally, for 5 minutes. Serve sprinkled with chives.

Prep Time: 35 Minutes

Cook Time: 35 Minutes

Servings: 4

Ingredients

- 1 pound Yukon Gold potatoes, peeled and cut into 1-inch pieces
- 3 tablespoons grapeseed oil or canola oil
- 1 large onion, diced
- 3 cloves garlic, minced
- 2 teaspoons curry powder
- ¾ teaspoon salt
- ¼ teaspoon cayenne pepper
- 1 (14 ounce) can no-salt-added diced tomatoes
- ¾ cup water, divided
- 1 (15 ounce) can low-sodium chickpeas, rinsed
- 1 cup frozen peas
- ½ teaspoon garam masala

Instructions

1. Bring 1 inch of water to a boil in a large pot fitted with a steamer basket. Add potatoes, cover and steam until tender, 6 to 8 minutes. Set the potatoes aside. Dry the pot.

2. Heat oil in the pot over medium-high heat. Add onion and cook, stirring often, until soft and translucent, 3 to 5 minutes. Add garlic, curry powder, salt and cayenne; cook, stirring constantly, for 1 minute. Stir in tomatoes and their juice; cook for 2 minutes. Transfer the mixture to a blender or food processor. Add 1/2 cup water and puree until smooth.

3. Return the puree to the pot. Pulse the remaining 1/4 cup water in the blender or food processor to rinse the sauce residue. Add to the pot along with the reserved potatoes, chickpeas, peas and garam masala. Cook, stirring often, until hot, about 5 minutes.

Prep Time: 25 Minutes

Cook Time: 1hrs 40 Minutes

Servings: 6

Ingredients

- 1 pound bone-in chicken drumsticks, skin removed
- 1 pound bone-in small chicken thighs, skin removed
- 1 teaspoon dried oregano
- 1 teaspoon garlic powder
- 1 teaspoon paprika
- ½ teaspoon ground pepper
- 1 teaspoon salt, divided
- 3 tablespoons extra-virgin olive oil
- 1 cup chopped red bell pepper
- 1 cup chopped white onion
- ¼ cup pitted green olives, sliced, plus more for garnish
- 3 large cloves garlic, finely chopped
- 4 cups low-sodium chicken broth
- 2 cups long-grain brown rice, rinsed
- ½ cup fire-roasted diced tomatoes
- 2 bay leaves

- ½ cup frozen green peas, thawed

Instructions

1. Combine chicken drumsticks, chicken thighs, oregano, garlic powder, paprika, pepper and 1/4 teaspoon salt in a medium bowl; stir well to coat.

2. Heat oil in a large high-sided pan or Dutch oven over medium heat. Add the chicken; cook, turning once, until golden brown on each side, about 8 minutes total. Transfer to a plate, leaving the juices in the pan. Add bell pepper, onion, olives and garlic to the pan; cook, stirring occasionally, until tender and fragrant, 3 to 4 minutes. Add broth, stirring to scrape up the brown bits on the bottom of the pan. Stir in rice, tomatoes, bay leaves and the remaining 3/4 teaspoon salt. Place the chicken on top of the rice; bring the mixture to a light boil. Reduce heat to medium-low; cook, half covered, until the rice is tender, most of the liquid is absorbed and an instant-read thermometer inserted in the thickest part of the chicken registers 165°F, about 60 minutes. Remove from heat. Add peas on top of the chicken and rice; cover and let stand until the liquid is absorbed, about 15 minutes. Discard the bay leaves

Prep Time: 30 Minutes

Cook Time: 45 Minutes

Servings: 4

Ingredients

- 3 tablespoons low-fat mayonnaise
- 1 teaspoon chili powder
- 2 medium sweet potatoes, peeled and cut into 1-inch cubes
- 4 teaspoons olive oil, divided
- ½ teaspoon salt, divided
- ¼ teaspoon ground pepper, divided
- 4 cups broccoli florets (8 oz.; 1 medium crown)
- 1 ¼ pounds salmon fillet, cut into 4 portions
- 2 limes, 1 zested and juiced, 1 cut into wedges for serving
- ¼ cup crumbled feta or cotija cheese
- ½ cup chopped fresh cilantro

Instructions

1. Preheat oven to 425 degrees F. Line a large rimmed baking sheet with foil and coat with cooking spray.
2. Combine mayonnaise and chili powder in a small bowl. Set aside.
3. Toss sweet potatoes with 2 tsp. oil, 1/4 tsp. salt, and 1/8 tsp. pepper in a medium bowl.
4. Spread on the prepared baking sheet. Roast for 15 minutes.
5. Meanwhile, toss broccoli with the remaining 2 tsp. oil, 1/4 tsp. salt, and 1/8 tsp. pepper in the same bowl.
6. Remove the baking sheet from oven. Stir the sweet potatoes and move them to the sides of the pan. Arrange salmon in the center of the pan and spread the broccoli on either side, among the sweet potatoes.
7. Spread 2 Tbsp. of the mayonnaise mixture over the salmon.
8. Bake until the sweet potatoes are tender and the salmon flakes easily with a fork, about 15 minutes.
9. Meanwhile, add lime zest and lime juice to the remaining 1 Tbsp. mayonnaise; mix well.
10. Divide the salmon among 4 plates and top with cheese and cilantro.

11. Divide the sweet potatoes and broccoli among the plates and drizzle with the lime-mayonnaise sauce. Serve with lime wedges and any remaining sauce.

Prep Time: 15 Minutes

Cook Time: 7hrs 35 Minutes

Servings: 6

Ingredients

- 1 pound dried cannellini beans, soaked overnight and drained
- 6 cups unsalted chicken broth
- 1 cup chopped yellow onion
- 1 cup sliced carrots
- 1 teaspoon finely chopped fresh rosemary
- 1 (4 ounce) Parmesan cheese rind plus 2/3 cup grated Parmesan, divided
- 2 bone-in chicken breasts (1 pound each)
- 4 cups chopped kale
- 1 tablespoon lemon juice
- ½ teaspoon kosher salt
- ½ teaspoon ground pepper
- 2 tablespoons extra-virgin olive oil
- ¼ cup flat-leaf parsley leaves

Instructions

1. Combine beans, broth, onion, carrots, rosemary and
   Parmesan rind in a 6-quart slow cooker. Top with
   chicken. Cover and cook on Low until the beans and
   vegetables are tender, 7 to 8 hours.
2. Transfer the chicken to a clean cutting board; let stand
   until cool enough to handle, about 10 minutes. Shred
   the chicken, discarding bones.
3. Return the chicken to the slow cooker and stir in kale.
   Cover and cook on High until the kale is tender, 20 to
   30 minutes.
4. Stir in lemon juice, salt and pepper; discard the
   Parmesan rind. Serve the stew drizzled with oil and
   sprinkled with Parmesan and parsley.

www.ingramcontent.com/pod-product-compliance
Lightning Source LLC
Chambersburg PA
CBHW051846250726
48659CB00006B/2050